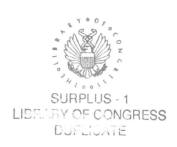

SURPLUS - 1
LIBRARY OF CONGRESS
DUPLICATE

D1374334

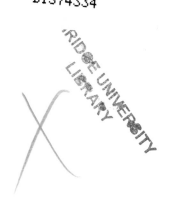

CAMBRIDGE UNIVERSITY
LIBRARY

Make Your Own Rainbows

MAKE YOUR OWN RAINBOWS

Louise Kendall

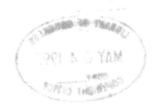

VANTAGE PRESS
New York • Los Angeles

RM
237.55
.K46
1991
C.3

33964

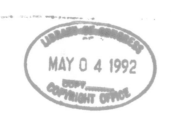

FIRST EDITION

All rights reserved, including the right of
reproduction in whole or in part in any form.

Copyright © 1991 by Louise Kendall

Published by Vantage Press, Inc.
516 West 34th Street, New York, New York 10001

Manufactured in the United States of America
ISBN: 0-533-09204-3

Library of Congress Catalog Card No.: 90-90216

1 2 3 4 5 6 7 8 9 0

Contents

Foreword

In this book I am giving you ideas and information that is meant to supplement your health care and guidance of your physician, not to replace it. Please do not attempt to embark on self-treatmemt of serious illness without their competent professional assistance. And I urge you to discuss any ideas you find here with your own physician.

I am telling you to the best of my ability, the honest facts that I have seen and experienced in my own life, and I hope that it will help you live a longer and happier life as you reach the twilight years of your life.

Living around my grandmother has made me aware of the danger of eating foods that are not good for you, and are downright poisonous to the body. And I have seen evidence that certain foods have improved the health of many patients.

Please check with your doctor, if you have any questions.

Introduction

This is a story about adding years of happiness to your life. I am writing this book out of love, respect, and a fond memory of a wonderful woman, my beloved grandmother, Doctor Frieda Christina Frederickson. She was known by her friends and patients as "Doctor Fred." She was years ahead of her time, and she tried to teach me everything she knew about being healthy and living a long and happy life. She would tell everyone to start early in life to eat the proper foods, and to exercise regularly. However, the bottom line was, "It's never too late to start taking care of your body."

I do not believe in plastic surgery, and I will submit to any examinations by any medical person or anyone else to prove that (1) I have never had plastic surgery, (2) my body is as firm and shapely as at the age of twenty, and (3) I have never had any children. I believe that the answer to many of our problems lie in the depths of the ocean. We all came from the ocean, and we need the life-giving nutrients the ocean provides. In the near future, we will all be amazed at the discoveries science will make from the ocean depths that will cure all our ills.

I am not a doctor, and I am not giving advice. All I want to do is tell you honestly, what I have seen with my own eyes, and heard, and experienced in my own life.

In this book, I will tell you all of my grandmother's secrets of how to live to be over a hundred years old, and enjoying every moment in a healthy body.

I will tell you why women live longer than men, and what you men out there can do about it, at any age. I will tell you of the patients she would take in with arthritis, in so much pain, they could hardly move. A week or so later, they would be walking around the house, and participating in the activities. A few weeks later, they would be out doing their own things.

I will tell you how, at age sixty-five, she looked like a thirty-year-old woman. And when she finally died, her face was still firm and beautiful. I also must add that she did not believe in plastic sugery. She would show how to get rid of, or prevent "platisma cording," commonly know as "turkey neck."

I will tell you what she told me about preservatives and additives in foods you eat. I will tell you what she told me about insecticides, and how we are being poisoned by them, and what we can do about it, to help, as much as we can, to keep out of harm's way.

I will tell you how I believe we are fooling ourselves about the AIDS virus. I believe it is much more contagious, and widespread than some institutions are willing to admit. More about this later.

I will tell you about what she would do with a few little white pills that she would buy at the corner drugstore that would cause a clean, painless and safe abortion for all the young ladies that would come to her, crying that they had been a "bad girl," or were unmarried and could not face their friends and neighbors. Doctor Fred would take them in and take care of them, most of the time, without any consideration of money. Some would stay overnight, in her big beautiful two-story home at 1235 East Filmore Street, in Phoenix, Arizona. The next morning they would be greeted in her big kitchen, with bacon and eggs, hot homemade biscuits and homemade preserves. Then they would be on their way to work, or wherever they had planned to go that day. Some girls would just stay for a few hours, and when it was over, they would leave. Some of the girls that had been there before, for the same reason, simply would go to the drugstore and buy the pills, and do it themselves, without consulting Doctor Fred. If the girls that stayed had no place to go, they would be welcome there, and in return would do a little work in the kitchen or laundry room, until Doctor Fred could help them get their lives together.

What a beautiful person my grandmother was. Her wise and thoughtful manner, her goodheartedness, and her understanding, kind, and generous ways made everyone love her, and want her somewhere in their lives.

A lot of the advice she gave was just common sense things, such as your own mother or grandmother would tell you a million times, like: "Eat your vegetables," or "Eat the peeling of the apple, (or potato) it's good for you." However, since the pesticides came on so strong, she would say, "Peel that apple or potato." The difference is, she would tell you why, and what to do about the pesticides, to protect your health.

Doctor Fred was a very important person in my life. She was very honest about everything, and she always said what she thought. She would answer all of my questions with straight answers. You always knew where you stood with her.

When I was a little girl, I remember it had been raining one day, and when the sun came out, there was a beautiful rainbow across the sky. After a while, the air dried and the rainbow went away. I started to cry, and she asked me what was the matter. I told her the rainbow went away. She proceeded to get the water hose, and positioned it so that a fine spray came down in the sunlight, and produced a very beautiful rainbow. I was so happy! Then my grandmother said to me, "Honey, in this life you have to make your own rainbows." I will never forget that moment. And I believe her. You have to get out there and do it, take charge of your life. Because no one is going to do it for you. Her confidence and faith,

AMRIDGE UNIVERSITY LIBRARY

along with her positive thinking and hope, have stayed with me, and I try to spread it around, and help everyone around me, in every way I can. Almost everyday, I use her advice, and remember many of her pearls of wisdom, which I will try to cover in this book.

Make Your Own Rainbows

Chapter 1

Zest for Life after the Big 100

You have probably heard the old joke about the man on his ninety-ninth birthday saying "If I had known I would live this long, I would have taken better care of myself." Well the purpose of this book is to give you the information you need to live a long and happy life, without the worry of poor health and outrageous medical bills, according to my grandmother, Doctor Fred.

On the following pages, I will tell you about the kinds of foods that I believe will have a beneficial effect on your health. If you are overweight, there are some tips on how to fool your body into feeling full on less food. Everyone that came to Doctor Fred to lose weight, did so, and kept it off easily. Doctor Fred was never over five or six pounds overweight. And when she realized it, she would cut back, and within a week or so she would be down to normal. I believe, however, that a few extra pounds on a healthy body are not harmful to your health. I also believe that there are a lot of worse things in food than sugar or salt. I think that some of the preservatives and additives in some foods alter the way the body handles the salt and sugar in our diets.

On the following pages, you will find information on the safe amounts of dietary allowances. As far as Doctor Fred was concerned, if a person eats the proper foods, and a great variety of vegetables, fruits, fish, coconut and pineapple, the only extra supplements you need are vitamin C, vitamin E, and cod liver oil, to maintain a healthy body.

Every day around five o'clock Doctor Fred would fix herself a Tanqueray Gibson. Except in the wintertime. When it was cold, she would opt for an eggnog, (Homemade, not that stuff you buy already made up.") or an Irish Coffee, made with one and one-half ounces Old Bushmill Irish Whiskey. She would say, "Celebrate every day of your life." Doctor Fred always felt that no matter what kind of day you have, it was a precious day to be living here on this Earth. She never had more than one drink, however. And she never smoked a cigarette. She said smoking makes a person old, wrinkled, and ugly. She said, "I don't mind being old, but I don't want to be wrinkled and ugly." It was simple for her to get anyone to stop smoking. She would have them, before they light up, take a bite out of grapefruit peeling, and chew it up. After that, when they took their first puff, they would say, "yuck!" and put that cigarette out! If you really want to quit, try it. It works.

Doctor Fred owned a beautiful car. It was big and shiny, and in perfect condition. However, she walked almost everywhere she went. She would start the car up every now and then, but she loved the exercise of walking. And it kept her agile in her later years. She was eighty-one when her mother died. That was a hard blow to her, as she was very close to her mother, and took very good care of her. But she blamed herself, because she was not at home, when her mother fell and hit her head. Doctor Fred was over a hundred years old when she herself died, and she worked every day right up to that day. She followed her own regimen, that she prescribed for her patients.

My grandmother was so dismayed and appalled by this country's "progress" regarding the use of additives, drugs, and pesticides on and in our food. However the one thing that discouraged her the most, and that she couldn't do anything about, was the news that she received one day about the pesticide residue that was found in honey. She was informed that many brands of honey were tested for pesticide contamination, and all were found to contain some traces of several different kinds of pesticides.

Evidently, the bees would carry the pesticides back to the hives, on their legs or wings, not knowing what it was. The pesticide had been sprayed on the blooms of the orange trees, clover, and wildflower, the three of her favorite kinds.

Doctor Fred would use the honey instead of sugar in all her baking of candies, cookies, fruit cakes, apple pies, and everything else that required sweetening. She would make the most delicious coleslaw dressing with a little honey, vinegar and mayonnaise. It was so good, she had to double her recipe, as everyone always asked for more, at mealtime. And her fruit cakes were so moist and delicious that everyone would beg for more. She would make dozens of fruit cakes around the holidays, and give them to friends and neighbors. She would make extra fruit cakes for stocking her pantry, but they didn't last long. We were all constantly sneaking in, and stealing them, so they were all gone soon after the holidays. Doctor Fred knew about it, and she was always flattered that we all appreciated her baking.

So one day, after she had given up on her beloved honey, she found this little old beekeeper that lived way out between Buckeye and Phoenix, Arizona. He had an orange grove, and right in the middle of it he kept about thirty hives of bees. The beekeeper's name was Larry. Larry was an old-fashioned farmer and did not use any kind of pesticides on his orange trees. He was a happy, good-natured little old man. He replied, when asked why he didn't use pesticides, "The bugs have to eat, too."

Well, I don't have to tell you how happy my grandmother was to find this treasure. Larry agreed to bring Doctor Fred's orders for two cases of honey, and five cases of oranges every two weeks, to the city, and deliver them to her door. She paid him well, and also threw in a little bit of good health care for him and his family, at no charge. This proved to be a long and happy relationship that lasted until Doctor Fred passed away. I will never forget how Larry sat down on the porch swing, at my grandmother's house and cried. It was a sad day for a great many people when "Doctor Fred" died.

Doctor Fred had a long and happy life, however, and she enjoyed every moment of it. I remember when I was young, she had a bicycle-built-for-two. And every day she would take her mother for a ride around the neighborhood. And sometimes I would be the lucky one. But then when her mother got older, and didn't feel like going, Doctor Fred retired the bicycle to her garage, and bought herself a regular one. She continued her rides around town three days a week, and went walking four days a week. This really kept her young and feeling good. Every morning before going on her exercise route, she would get a tray of ice cubes, drop them in the bathroom sink, fill the basin with water and soak her face in the ice water. She would do this for several minutes, taking deep breaths in between soaks. This made her face very firm, over the years, and she stayed beautiful and young-looking all her life. Doctor Fred would advise all the girls against putting hot water on their faces. She said never never never to put hot water on your face! Put cold water only. She said hot water makes the skin sag. Cold water makes it firm and solid. And she was living proof.

Sometimes while on her exercise route, Doctor Fred would jog or run rather than walk. Many mornings some of the girls would accompany her. Doctor Fred would advise them to wear a good strong bra while exercising. Because while jumping up and down running, the breast muscles would weaken, and the breasts would drop down several inches. One girl had a lovely figure, and she never wore a bra while

4

jogging. Over time, her breasts dropped down, and made her look like an older woman. She was sorry that she had not taken Doctor Fred's advice, because she was a young woman and had lost her young figure.

Doctor Fred was adamant about wearing the proper shoes, too. If you don't have proper shoes for exercising, a great deal of harm can be done to the feet. So be sure that you have sturdy, proper fitting lace-up shoes before you go jogging, running, or walking. I usually use two pairs of socks. I find they cushion my step and are more comfortable for me. Sometimes I run, and sometimes I walk. Sometimes I jog, and sometimes I ride my bicycle. It all depends on how I feel that particular day. But I try to do some exercising every day.

I have never really been overweight in my life, and it is a miracle, considering all the good foods I was exposed to during my life. Sometimes, however, I will put on a few extra pounds around the holidays. So I start cutting back. I drink a lot of water. Just before I drink a glass of fruit juice, I drink a glass or so of cold water. When I finish the fruit juice, I feel as if I have had two or three glasses of fruit juice. Before each meal, I eat a half of an apple, or one small whole apple. Then I drink a glass of buttermilk. By the time I get half through the meal, I am completely satisfied. Within one week, I am back down to my regular weight.

The secret to weight loss is keeping the mind occupied, just as Doctor Fred would say. Get involved with something that interests you. You will forget all about food. The reason many people overeat is because they are bored. So do something exciting. There are a lot of things to do that are not expensive, or that cost nothing at all. The library would be a good place to start. Go in and look up your favorite subject. You can get a lot of ideas there. And once you get involved, you will forget about food. As an example, since I have started writing this book, I have lost five pounds. And I never had weight loss in mind when I started it. I get in here in my little cubbyhole with my trusty old typewriter, and I forget about eating. All at once, I look up, and it's dark outside. Since I forget to eat, I am careful to take my vitamins and minerals every day.

I have had remarkably good health all my life, and I am very grateful to God that He blessed me with it. Oh, sometimes, when I have had a bad day, I feel about fifty years old, but most of the time I feel about thirty-something.

I try to take my grandmother's advice and think young. It does help. I always try to look at the bright side of everything. As they always say, "If life gives you a lemon, make lemonade with it." Well, I have had a few lemons all right. But I have too much to be grateful for to let it get me down.

My grandmother also had a good sense of humor. She would say things like, "If it don't fit, force it." or "Eat your vegetables, they are good for your liver. You want to be along liver, don't you?" Or she would tell of the doctor examining a business tycoon: "Contrary to what the union says, your heart IS in the right place." I have heard her say: "Success covers a multitude of blunders." "Nothing is so permanent as something temporary." "If bankers can count, how come they have eight windows and only three tellers?" "He was so popular nobody could stand him." "One doctor to another: 'When you can't guess what's ailing a man, just ask his wife.' " And, "I've never had a guilty conscience. The only thing I ever did at night that I was sorry for in the morning was set the alarm clock."

I always use Alpha Beta brand of mayonnaise. It is the only brand that I have found that is completely without artificial preservatives and has the delicious and delicate flavor of real mayonnaise. I have searched far and wide, and I have not found any thing that would compare with Alpha Beta Brand. And I am very grateful to Alpha Beta markets for offering this product to their customers. And I am surprised at the other big name brands, that charge more money for their mayonnaise, and continue to add all the preservatives in it. I would gladly pay Alpha Beta more money for their brand, if I had to in order to keep their brand pure as it is. (But don't tell them that!)

For Thanksgiving, my grandmother would bake the turkey with a special honey basting sauce that made the turkey moist and so delicious it would make your taste buds jump up and down. And her honied ham and chicken—mmmm good. I could go on and on.

In the summer months we would drag out the old ice-cream maker and make ice cream from my grandmothers favorite recipes. If you have never had ice cream made with honey instead of sugar, you don't know what you have missed. Her honey-vanilla, honey-pineapple and honey-peach were outstanding. My favorite was her honey-lemon. It was heavenly. No one could refuse a second helping, but most of the time it was third or fourth helpings. Another thing I loved to eat were her honey-baked apples. All these things that she would make with honey were so mouth watering. It's no wonder everyone spent so much of our time in the kitchen. It was a magical place.

Another favorite room to hang out in was her parlor. Doctor Fred had a big beautiful piano there. And in the evenings, she would go in and sit down at the piano, and play everyone's requests. And most of us would sing along until time for bed. What a fortunate life I had.

My parents were divorced, and consequently I spent a good deal of time with my grandmother. And believe me, I loved every moment of it. I was very lucky, and I knew it at the time, and was very grateful to her. However, the time would come when I would realize a more deeply profound gratitude.

When I moved to Los Angeles, in the 1950s, I was exposed to a very different side of life. I had gone to visit my older brother in Los Angeles from time to time over the years, but it was not the same as living there. I saw things that I had never seen before. The homeless, which made me sad. The crime. The smog—back home I never saw smog. The traffic. I'll never forget the first time I drove on the freeways. My heart was in my throat all the while. I was scared to death. The first time I ever got a traffic ticket was on the San Bernadino freeway, for going too slow. Heck, I was from the country, I was used to dirt roads, cow trails. What did I know? Then all at once all these cars were passing me so quickly, and so close to me! The noise alone scared the daylights out of me. I stayed on the sidestreets from then on, for a long time.

One day I was standing at an upstairs window, at my brother's home, marveling at the sights of the big city. Along came a man with a red and white cane. He was waving the cane back and forth in front of him. I asked my brother what he was doing that for. My brother said, "Honey, that man is blind." I was in a state of shock. I had never seen a blind person before. As I watched him, tears came to my eyes. I told my brother that I wanted to do down and help him. I don't know what I was going to do, I just knew that he needed help of some kind. My brother explained to me that you can't just go up to a person and try to help them. He told me that some people are very proud, and that some people might be offended if I approached them. He said that there were many many people like that in Los Angeles. And that there were people in wheelchairs, and worse.

He said, "If you want to help people like that, get a good job, and donate money to them, and go down to the mission, and donate your time to help them out. But you can't just go up to a person on the street and stop them. They might think you are going to hurt them, or rob them."

So, I took his advice. My brother, Bob, God love him, is such a good person, and he has a heart of gold.

It was Bob that everyone would call on when they needed help of any kind. He was always, and still is, kind, gentle, goodhearted and honest. He will come to anyone's aid, anytime. Old, young, black, white, rich or poor. He spent four years in the Navy. And has recently retired from the phone company. When he came home from the Navy, he went directly to Los Angeles, and to work for the phone company. So I didn't spend as much time with him as I would have liked. But he was always there for me when I needed him. Always considerate of the other person's feelings and thoughtful about birthdays, anniversaries, and holidays, he is the perfect brother. Once for Christmas I got him a lovely Arnold Palmer sweater. Bob looked at it, and said, in all sincerity, "Gosh it's beautiful. And I didn't even know he could knit."

I remember when my brother was a young boy back in Arizona. A little dog had been hit by a car, and his hind leg had been injured. My brother, Bob picked the dog up, and cradled it in his arms and using only one hand, rode his bicycle home, and took care of the little dog. He put a bandage on the dog's leg, and fed it. And for several weeks, everywhere Bob went, you could see him carrying that little dog around on his bicycle. It was so cute. And so typical of my big brother.

My brother recently sold his home in North Hollywood and moved to Canoga Park. It's little farther away, but still convenient to see him often. And just a phone call away. It's nice to get together once in a while, to talk about the good old days.

Sometimes I would ride my horse to school, rather than go on the bus. One day my girlfriend and I decided to ride double-saddle on my horse to school. We were almost to school when the school bus came along, and just at that time, the saddle, which had not been cinched tightly enough started to slide down to the horse's stomach and we both fell off. Thank God, the ground was sandy and soft, so we didn't get hurt. But you should have heard the laughing, screaming, and yelling that came from the school bus. We got the saddle back on the horse, cinched it properly, and continued on to school. However, our pride was definitely bruised. The other students teased us something awful for weeks after that. We thought we would never get over the embarrassment. Subsequently, my brother showed me how to cinch a horse, when riding double-saddle, so it would not come loose. I had no further problems after that. Bob, I love you.

Chapter 2

Why Women Live Longer than Men

This is the advice Doctor Fred would give the male patients, all of whom I found lived to be over one hundred years old. And all were running every day and enjoying their lives right up to the day they died.

The reason, according to Doctor Fred, that men don't live as long as women, is because women have their menstrual cycles. This loss of blood every month forces the body to replace the lost blood with new blood and consequently revives the old blood. Women also have babies, which causes more loss of blood. And more blood is replaced by new blood. Doctor Fred would joke to the men, "If you want to live longer, start having babies."

But seriously, she would have all the men patients go down to the Red Cross, and donate blood every two months. This would compensate for the nonloss of blood during their lifetime. She would have all her male patients on a regular regimen, of proper diet: no preservatives of any kind, and pesticide free; lots of fresh fruits and vegetables, especially pineapple, coconut, apples, figs and dates; skim milk, fish and oysters; lemonade and lots of water; one and one-half ounces of whiskey per day; lots of walking or running, and eye exercises.

For about five minutes a day, she would sit the patients down, and have them roll their eyes around, making circles as large as they could. After a while many found they didn't need their glasses any longer. At the end of the day, she would give them one tablespoonful of apple-cider vinegar, mixed with a glass of cold water. But above all, she would instill positive thinking, faith, confidence, mind over matter, and hope always for a better tomorrow.

Chapter 3

An Open Letter to President Bush

Dear President Bush:

Every now and then, I hear of some influential person making the statement that America's children suffer from malnutrition, especially the ones on welfare, on the poverty level. They rant on and on, about how the President should throw more and more money at it, and it will go away. They are constantly asking you for more money, to solve the problem of people on welfare.

Well I believe that the children suffer from malnutrition, but no matter how much money you give them, it will not solve the problem. The reason I say this, is because I have made a study of how the welfare mothers spend their food stamps. I have stood in endless lines in supermarkets around the country, and observed what the mothers were buying with their food stamps. I saw endless piles of cookies, candy, cakes, ice cream, potato chips and carts piled high with sodapop of all kinds. These poor children have no choice, they have to eat what their mothers bring into the house. Most of the children don't know any better, and even if they did, they have no choice. Besides, it tastes good to them. Very seldom did I see any vegetables, rice, beans or fresh fruit in their carts. I believe these food stamps should only be good for the wholesome foods that contain the nutritious value that these people need. Food stamps are not accepted for beer, liquor, wine, or cigarettes. Why should they be accepted for junk food, which is full of empty calories and no nutrition? If you could make the stamps good only for bread, milk, vegetables, fresh fruit, rice, beans, cereal, any canned foods and pasta, it would force the mothers to buy only wholesome foods for their families and do a little home cooking, rather than eating constantly out of bags. I have interviewed many of the women on welfare, and most of them told me that they hate to cook, and it is easier for them, if the kids grab a bag of potato chips and a Coke, and fall in front of the television set.

Well, I myself could afford to eat out in a restaurant every day of the week, if I wanted to. But I hardly ever eat out. I buy the good things and bring them home and cook for my loved one and myself, and this way I know exactly what we are eating, and enjoy the health the nutritious food gives us. It is not going to hurt these women on welfare to cook a decent meal for their families.

Mr. President, please change the rules on the food stamps. We don't need more money, we need some hard love. And we will have a healthier happier bunch of kids growing up, and fewer doctor bills.

God Bless you, Mr. President, and I want you to know that you have our prayers to ask God to help guide you along your very difficult and complex path. We are all behind you all the way, And you have our undying love and support in everything you do.

Chapter 4

Send Them to Camp

When I went home for a visit one time, I took a copy of the *Los Angeles Times* with me. My grandmother picked it up and read it. There were a lot of stories about gang violence. One story was about a youth that had been picked up by the police at three o'clock in the morning for fighting with three other youths in the town of East Los Angeles. My grandmother asked me, "What in the world are these kids doing out on the streets at three o'clock in the morning?" I told her that it was very common to see gang members out on the streets in the early morning hours. She said, "Don't you know that these kids are screaming for discipline, crying out for guidance? Where are their parents?" She told me that in her day the city would set a curfew, and any child caught loitering on the streets were sent to the CC (Civilian Conservation) Camps. There they would get a good education, discipline, guidance, and a respect for authority. The Camps made good citiznes out of these young men that refused to go to school on their own. I sincerely believe this is a wonderful solution to the gang problems.

If these kids have a full day of study and exercise, they would be so tired, the last thing on their minds would be to hang around street corners at three o'clock in the morning. They would be so grateful for a bed and a nice soft pillow at that hour. And the best part of all, it would get them away from the drug scene and make good men out of them. I have talked to all my friends and neighbors about this and they all agree the U.S. should start up the CC Camps once again. It would make a big difference, and end the gang problems in Los Angeles, as well as the rest of the nation.

Chapter 5

Safe Abortion

Doctor Fred believed that daily estrogen tablets taken after menopause are an effective means of slowing or preventing bone deterioration, also known as osteoporosis, a bone loss that can deform or cripple older women. She said the estrogen therapy was to be used in addition to regular regimen of a proper high calcium diet, and lots of exercise. Doctor Fred treated all her women patients after menopause with estrogen. She knew thirty or forty years ago that this helped to prevent bone deterioration. As I said before, she was ahead of her time. She warned against taking too much, however. Some doctors today prescribe up to 10 mg. or more. Doctor Fred would prescribe the lowest doses consisting of 0.3 premarin once a day for twenty-five days. Then one tablet of 2 mg. provera per day for five days. She believed a larger dose of provera (medroxyprogesterone) would cause problems such as thinning of the hair, and more growth of facial hair, among other things. Many women taking the larger doses of provera have noticed a heavy growth of facial hair, and also a tendency to cancer. Doctor Fred said, "No one needs that much."

Doctor Fred believed that "toxic shock syndrome" was caused not by the tampons used, but by the length of time they were allowed to remain in the vagina. Some women would forget they had them in, and leave it in there for weeks. She treated one lady for toxic shock syndrome, and she found out the patient had forgotten to remove the last tampon she had used. She didn't realize it until her next period came

17

around, and she was very ill. Doctor Fred removed the old tampon and pulled her through it. The woman recovered! However, Doctor Fred admonished her against leaving any tampon in for more than a few hours, and to advise her to take a douche after her period. Doctor Fred was aware of the problems of the tampons, and the lawsuits. However, she said it was not the fault of the tampons. It was lack of proper hygiene. One girl came to see Doctor Fred complaining of pains in her abdomen. Doctor Fred examined her, and found nine tampons inside her vagina. Every time the girl would notice traces of blood on her panties, she would put in another tampon.

"What we need here is more education," said Doctor Fred. She was all for having classes taught in school, so that this kind of thing would never happen again. The girl had a high fever, and was half out of her mind. With a lot of apple-cider douches, megadoses of vitamin C, along with cold baths and pineapple juice, apple juice, coconut juice and grapefruit juice, and her medication, Doctor Fred pulled her through.

When she left, she was the picture of health, but heaven only knows what would have happened, if the girl had not come to Doctor Fred when she did. Doctor Fred sat the girl down and explained all about the menstrual cycle, what causes it, what it is for, and how to handle it. Doctor Fred said every girl should know all about this subject by the time they start menstruating.

Doctor Fred also said, "The best and safest birth control method there is, is the word no! Especially for young unmarried girls."

This is the advice Doctor Fred gave for a clean, fast, painless, easy abortion.

"In preparation for this event, the day before, be sure to take all your regular vitamins and minerals, which I have already outlined in the past. Plus take about one thousand mg. extra, of vitamin C. Do not eat anything on the morning of the abortion, but do take another tablet of one thousand mg. vitamin C. Get the things you will need together, such as a good book or sewing. Some women just watch television. Above all get comfortable."

Doctor Fred would start off explaining how important timing is in this procedure. "After you miss your first period, you count twenty-eight days from the first day of your last period. This is when your period should have started. Then you count twenty-eight days from this day. For example, If the last period you missed was due on the tenth of November, you count twenty-eight days, which would put you at December 8. This is the day you start. Go down to the nearest drug store, and purchase a bottle of quinine tablets.

"First you take three tablets with water, wait one half hour. Then take three more tablets. Wait one hour. Take two more tablets. Wait one hour. Most women will have started their period by this time. If nothing happens, however, take two more tablets. Wait one hour more. Take two more tablets. Do not take more than twelve tablets total. When you feel your period coming, go to the bathroom, clean up, take a nice shower, and put on a regular Kotex. Lie down and rest and finish that book, or have a nice lunch. The only side effects you will notice will be a slight ringing in your ears. This will fade away within an hour or so. Be sure to resume your regular healthy diet and the vitamin supplement I have given you earlier."

As I said before, some women do this while at work or while at their regular activities. One girl that used to work with me had three children, and didn't want anymore. So she would buy the pills and take them while at work. One day she said, "Oh, I just aborted, I have to get some Kotex, would you watch my station?" I said sure I would. And a few minutes later she came back and resumed her job, as if nothing had happened. I have seen this happen over and over again. So I believe it is safe and easy and convenient.

The strength quinine tablets that Doctor Fred advised the girls to take was 350 mg., which can be purchased without a prescription.

The reason some girls would get their own pills, and not consult Doctor Fred, was because they were embarrassed. When a girl came to her she would help them out of their situation, but not without a stern lecture. Doctor Fred would explain everything about pregnancy, birth control, and the risks of disease. She didn't mind at all helping a girl out of a bad situation the first time, because anyone can make a mistake. However, if the same girl came to her again, for the same reason, Doctor Fred would be very cross with her, because the girl had not learned her lesson. Doctor Fred would tell them, "The best birth control in the world is the word no!" The last thing she would say to them, when they left the house was, "You be a good girl now!"

Chapter 6

High Density Lipoprotein

High density lipoprotein (HDL) acts as a scavenger, transporting fatty substances to the liver where they are excreted. Therefore, the higher HDL level a person has, the lower the risk of coronary artery disease. Doctor Fred would advise patients to take vigorous exercise and moderate amounts of alcohol to elevate their HDL levels.

The more I read and learn about health and disease, the more I am convinced of the wisdom of the teachings of my grandmother, Doctor Fred. Every book and every article I read lately is saying the same things that she taught me years and years ago. She was adamant about exercise, not smoking and the moderate use of alcohol. She warned, however against taking more than one or two drinks a day. There are certain foods she would swear by. In this chapter you will find a list of them. She would say, "If you can, eat the vegetables raw. If you cook them, it is a sin to overcook them. Better undercooked."

She would keep two large jars of water in the refrigerator, with a lemon squeezed in each one, and she would drink this when she wanted water. When she wanted something sweet, she would drink fruit juices. She never bought soda pop of any kind. She would say the soda pop had too much artificial flavoring, coloring, and preservatives to suit her. I have read the labels on the soda pop, and she was right. I believe she was right, also, when she said that these additives will harm the immune system.

It is good to cut down on cholesterol, but I think the body needs a certain amount, and some people are overreacting, and cutting out foods that the body needs, like eggs and dairy products, unnecessarily. When patients would come to Doctor Fred with high levels of cholesterol Doctor Fred would start giving them 50 milligrams of niacin with each meal. Right away, their cholesterol levels dropped about 50 points. Then Doctor Fred would have them on her regular regimen, with proper diet, and exercise, and one and one-half ounces of alcohol per day, and then she would discontinue the niacin. This therapy worked on all her patients.*

The safe amount of selenium intake is 150 micrograms a day. And it is important to include this in your diet. Also use biotin, a member of the vitamin B complex. A safe amount of biotin would be 200 micrograms a day. Eating raw egg whites prevents the body from absorbing biotin. This is the reason Doctor Fred cautioned against eating raw egg whites. Always cook them. A proper amount of biotin also prevents baldness, or loss of hair. However again, do not overdo it and take too much of any supplement. Talk to your own doctor, and discuss vitamin supplements with him or her so you will feel confident about your health.

For your information, I have discovered a "Food Hot Line," which you can call if you have any questions about food, or restaurants, on the food industry. There is no charge for the service. The number to call is (213) 900-2111. I have not called it, but they claim to have the answers to any questions.

Men have a need for exercise because it will prevent high blood pressure in most cases, and lower it also. After a three-

---

*These patients continued to have a cholesterol level of 150, for the rest of their lives, and remained healthy and happy until over a hundred years old.

month program of regular twenty-minute fast-paced workouts on a stationary bicycle the blood pressure will go down from ten to fifty points. You can walk away or run away from high blood pressure.

If you are watching your weight, it is important to know that because fat is more than twice as rich in calories as carbohydrates and protein, you can eat a lot of the good low-fat foods before you meet your calorie quota. You don't have to eat a lot less, you have to eat more carefully. Be sure and get a lot of oysters and water-packed tuna. Also skim milk, yogurt and low-fat cottage cheese. High blood pressure can be controlled without drugs. Nutrition is the key.

Magnesium is important because it helps keep the tiny blood components called platelets from clumping together and blocking blood vessels. It will also not only help men avoid a heart attack but survive one should it occur. So eat those oysters and fish, as they are a good source of magnesium. They are also a good source of zinc. Zinc can prevent toxic metals like cadmium and lead from accumulating in the body. The RDA for zinc is fifteen mg. per day.

Pectin is a water-soluable fiber that helps to control cholesterol in the body. A good source of pectin and delightful to eat are apples, oranges, pears, carrots, and beets.

Chapter 7

Odds and Ends

Don't believe everything you read in advertising. Here are a few examples of advertising that you should be aware of. Take "sugarless gum." It may help you avoid tooth decay, but don't kid yourself that you are ingesting fewer calories. Chances are you're consuming just as many as if you chewed sugared gum. The culprit in this case is a substance called "sorbitol," a natural sweetener that contains as many calories as sugar. Plenty of other foods and beverages labeled "sugar-free" can have a lot of sugar-like calories.

Or take non-dairy creamers. "Nondairy" means anything but nonsaturated. You should know that most nondairy creamers contain a great deal of coconut oil, which is more saturated than milkfat, although it does not contain cholesterol.

Or take fiber supplements. While more people have become concerned about the amount of fiber in their diets, not many know that even if you ate an entire bottle of most self-billed high-fiber pills, you wouldn't get the fiber available in a bowl of strawberries.

Or vitamins. Have you ever heard about the new vitamin B-32? If you have, you've heard wrong. There is no such thing as B-32!

Here in Southern California, with the earthquakes, and possibility of a water shortage, and needing all the water you can get, instead of putting bricks in your toilet tank, as some city personnel suggested, in order to save water, instead put in clean jars or bottles full of water, with tight fitting lids, and you will have water when you need it.

Let's talk about toilet paper. I believe toilet paper that is colored or has patterns on it should be banned. Yes it is pretty, and it brightens up a bathroom. But the dyes in it are helping to destroy the ecology, and it could pose a danger to some people, especially the elderly. I know of a lady who used a pink colored toilet paper with red roses on it. She had a medical problem that she was not aware of. Every time she went to the toilet, there was a bloody discharge. Because of the color of the toilet paper, the blood went unnoticed. She thought the red color was from the toilet paper. Consequently, she did not go to the doctor as soon as she should have. If the toilet paper had been pure white, she would have noticed the blood, and gone to her doctor sooner. Think about it.

Never never never stand over the top of a gas stove, and breathe the unburned fumes of gas, when you are lighting the stove. And never never never breathe the fumes of gasoline, when you are filling your gas tank. These fumes can cause damage to your lungs, even in very small amounts.

Always use apple cider or rice vinegar, for cooking or consuming. It is much better for you and you should have some of it every day. The white kind of vinegar is only good for cleaning or bleaching.

When taking vitamin and mineral tablets, always break them up in your mouth, a little, or chew them somewhat, because otherwise the tablet will pass on through your body, and not dissolve, consequently depriving the body of the nutrition.

Always keep a lot of plants around the house. They provide oxygen, and help keep the household air clean and fresh. If you have a microwave oven, in the kitchen, keep a plant near it, because the plant will be the first to tell you if your microwave oven has a leak. If it is leaking microwaves, which are dangerous to your health, the plant will shrivel up and die.

Before you start your holiday cooking, check your spice rack. Be sure that all your spices are fresh, because not only are old, stale spices not good for you, they have lost their flavor and zest.

Doctor Fred thought toothpaste should be banned. She brushed her teeth with baking soda. She had all her own teeth all her life, and she would brag to us when she would have a checkup. She thought that the chemicals in toothpaste were very harmful if swallowed, even in very small amounts, especially for children. There was the possibility a child would swallow greater amounts of it. She said that if the child swallowed great amounts of baking soda it would not harm him or her.

Most of the brands of toothpaste contain: Sodium monofluorophosphate, dicalcium phosphate, dihydrate, glycerin, sodium lauryl sulfate, cellulose gum, sodium benzoate, tetrasodium pyrophosphate, and sodium saccharin.

Some of these chemicals are accumulative in our bodies. So in a year's time, all these chemicals added to a small amount of food additives, added to a small amount of pesticides, added to a small amount of preservatives and added to a small amount of hormones, each day, with the definite possibility of interaction of the chemicals, you have a potent little cocktail.

Doctor Fred advised all her patients to use baking soda to brush their teeth with, and if they should swallow some of it, it would be good for the stomach. It is natural and harmless if swallowed.

We believe there is plenty of fluoride in our drinking water and the baking soda does as good a job as toothpaste.

Chapter 8

Body Shapes

Doctor Fred thought that a few extra pounds could be a source of emotional distress. But in terms of your health, all fat deposits are not the same. You are at greater risk if you look like an apple than if you look like a pear. Pear-shaped persons, who store fat in their thighs and hips, can be moderately overweight and still not develop health problems related to obesity. People who gain weight primarily in their lower body probably don't have any greater health risks than those who are not overweight at all.

Apple-shaped men and women however, deposit fat around the abdomen. Even a few extra pounds there may heighten your risk of heart disease, diabetes, and high blood pressure. If you have an apple-shaped body, make special efforts to increase physical activity and follow a reduced-fat diet. Shedding the extra pounds will reduce obesity-related health risks. A sensible approach to weight control will help you enjoy the fruits of good health.

Chapter 9

Turkey Neck

Platisma cording, commonly known as turkey neck, occurs when the skin on the neck underneath the chin loses its elasticity and hangs down, giving the profile a completely different appearance from that of the person's younger years. It tends to make the person look older. Gravity is mostly to blame for this condition.

The best thing to do is to prevent this from happening. And you have to start while you are young. However, most of us don't even notice it until the condition is pretty well along. The method to prevent this condition is the same as to cure it. The main thing to remember is the sooner you start, the better chance you have of reversing this undesirable effect of gravity on your profile.

Once again, the answer is exercise. First of all, you have to find a place where no one can see you do this exercise, because they will surely think you have gone stark crazy. When you get all comfortable and seated behind locked doors, you tilt your head back, as far as you can, jut out your chin, and pull as hard as you can. Pulling your chin up as far as you can, and with your back straight, try to close your teeth, as if chewing. If you have done it right, with your head back far enough, you will have a hard time closing your teeth together. But force them up and down, as if chewing. You should feel the pull on the neck muscles. Then lean back a little, and you will feel it even more. It will feel good. Then after a few minutes bring the head down, rest a few seconds, then repeat.

Do this every day, and in about a week, do it in front of a mirror. You will notice the difference right away, if the condition is not too far advanced. The further advanced the condition, the longer it will take to tighten up the muscles, but it feels so good, once you start, you will do it regularly.

In order to hasten the results, you can put your hand, with four fingers together, and press the forefinger into the neck just above the Adam's apple, when the teeth are apart, then release as you try to close, and pull up on your chin. You will have your head back as far as you can, you will be jutting your chin out, trying to close your teeth. The side of your forefinger will be placed where the chin and the neck meet. You will open your teeth, as you press in on your throat, and you will release your hand, as you make the chewing motion of closing your teeth. All the while, your head will be as far back as you can lean. The length of time it will take you to get the desired results will depend on the amount of time you spend doing the exercise.

It also helps to think happy thoughts, while doing this exercise. Think how beautiful, or handsome you will be without that turkey neck. It also helps if you turn on a radio and find some nice romantic music to go along with your happy thoughts.

This exercise is one that you will enjoy doing, because it feels so good to be using these muscles that have been neglected for so long.

Chapter 10

Eating Your Way to Good Health

The old expression, "You are what you eat," is one that should not be forgotten, especially when deciding where and what to eat. Presently, more than 50 percent of Americans' food budget is spent in restaurants and fast food places, as opposed to 29 percent ten years ago. Could this be one of the reasons that the instances of malnutrition-related diseases are increasing? The average American consumes more than 400 soft drinks (38 gallons) per year. Just think of the food coloring, additives and preservatives that are accumulating in the system, just from the beverage alone, not to mention the amounts contained in the food we eat. No wonder our immune systems are in a state of shock.

The manufacturers are flooding the markets with foods that are processed and full of preservatives, additives, chemicals, and colorings that are poisonous to our bodies, and in some cases have caused death. And add to that the pesticides and hormones used even before the foods get to the processors, that are such a threat to the health of all Americans. We have to do something about it as quickly as possible!

Because of all the new viruses and diseases that are being brought to this country lately, we are going to have to build up our immune systems in order to fight them off. And we are going to have to start today. It is a matter of life or death. My intention with this book is to help you achieve this goal, and make you aware of the dangers of some of the foods that we tend to take for granted.

The health superstars: Mushrooms. Some mushrooms stimulate the immune system and benefit the heart. They are known in China as "The Chinese God of Longevity." Like beans, mushrooms are low in certain amino acids. A fresh pound has only 125 calories. They are not to be eaten raw, however. Cooking breaks down the cell walls and destroys any toxins.

Fish: All kinds. Oysters were given to patients complaining of dry mouth, and not enough tears in the eyes to move them comfortably. They were completely cured and had no further problems when adding two ounces or more per day of canned oysters to their diet. When the oysters were discontinued the dry mouth and dry eyes syndrome returned.

Nuts: All kinds. Especially peanuts and peanut butter— the brands that contain no preservatives. (Read the labels, girls.)

Bran and Oat Bran	Beans and Kidney Beans
Dried Figs	Bananas
Green Peas	Raisins
Coconuts	Pineapples
Carrots	Broccoli and Cauliflower
Soybeans	Rice
Apples and Apple Juice	Oranges and Grapefruit

Vinegar (apple cider or rice only)
Onions and Garlic
Milk and Milk Products
Eggs (Never eat raw eggs. Always cook them.)
Grapes and Grape Juice

One of Grandma's favorite things to cook, was stuffed celery. She would bake it with bread crumbs, the same way she would make the dressing for chicken or turkey. We liked

31

it so much, she had to cook three or four large stalks at a time.

If you like potatoes with lots of butter on them, and want to cut down on calories, try Huston's Yukon Gold Potatoes. They come with the butter built into them. Their creamy yellow flesh and rich buttery taste make high-fat additions seem superfluous. Yet they contain no fat whatsoever. They are also good sources of dietary fiber, potassium and vitamin C. One medium Yukon Gold potato (150 grams) contains 110 calories, 3 grams of protein and 23 grams of carbohydrate. Boil the potato and drain the liquid. Place back in the pot over low heat. Mash the potatoes, adding ½ cup buttermilk until very smooth, add salt, pepper and chives. Mix well. Delicious.

If you have a weight problem, which most of us do at some time or another, it may help you to know what Doctor Fred thought on the subject. She said sometimes, when our mind is hungry, we feed our mouths instead. If you are bored, sit down, and think of the thing you like most to do, the thing that interests you the most. Then get involved in it. If it is sewing, then start a regular sewing bee. If it is painting, start getting your materials together. Make time for the things you want to do. If it is sky diving, surfing, exploring, hang gliding or something else that is hard to do, go to the library and study up on the subject, read books on the subject, get involved with what you love to do. Believe me, you will forget about food. You will be feeding your mind rather than over-feeding your body.

Chapter 11

Cancer Prevention Tips

This is the advice Doctor Fred would give regarding cancer prevention. And she lived and breathed her own advice. She said if it was good enough for her patients, it was good enough for her. Here goes: Don't smoke or use any tobacco in any form. Eat food low in fat. Include fresh fruits, vegetables and whole grains, apple cider vinegar, pineapples, oysters and low-fat milk in your diet. If you drink alcoholic beverages, do so in moderation. Avoid unnecessary X rays. Avoid too much sunlight; wear protective clothing; use sun screens. Keep yourself safe on the job by using protective devices (respirators, protective clothing.) Do not eat any preservatives, food dyes, or pesticides. Read the labels on food products, and wash fruits and vegetables thoroughly, or peel the outer layer off, as it contains the pesticides. Drink as much water as frequently as you can. Maintain a regular schedule for mealtime. Avoid fried foods. Have your meals with friends or family and in a pleasant atmosphere. Remain active, get plenty of exercise. This way, even if you do get the cancer virus, your immune system will be able to fight it, and you can lick it.

Doctor Fred was very particular about the restaurants she would go to. She maintained that old or rancid grease was very harmful to the immune system. A lot of restaurants use stale grease to cook their food in and rancid butter to butter their toast with. Also she was aware of the sulfites, preservatives, and food colors all restaurants used. She would only go out about three times a year to have dinner. Not that she could not afford it, she just didn't trust them. She would advise everyone to stay away from the "greasy spoons," and to cook at home, where you have control over the things you put in your body. She said that the preservatives and additives in food helped to bind the cholesterol to the arteries, giving us one more reason to eliminate them from our diets. Sulfites and some drugs can destroy the immune system. Everyone should stay away from them. Don't take any drugs unless they are prescribed by your physician.

You have to make sure that most of your diet consists of "nutrient defense foods." Inadequate amounts of certain vitamins and minerals can cause serious problems in older people. Vitamin B-6 requirements are higher for people over sixty. They also need to meet their needs for zinc and vitamin B-2, which helps release energy from carbohydrates, proteins, and fats, and aids in the maintenance of mucous membranes. Sufficient amounts of vitamin D are necessary for proper calcium absorption. Lots of onions and garlic should be continued in the diets of older people. If you start getting into good nutritional and exercise habits, you will be more optimistic and have a more positive attitude and feel much better into the twilight years.

Chapter 12

Feeding the Body's Immune System

As everyone is aware nowadays of the importance of the function of the immune system, and the protection and preservation of it because of the AIDS epidemic, I want to share what Doctor Fred told me about it. First of all she said that most viruses have a lot in common. They all like a nice warm and moist place to multiply. A virus cannot tell if it is in a man, woman, or child. She said that all viruses are contagious and can be transmitted the same way the cold virus is spread. I believe that we have a monster on our hands here in the United States with the AIDS virus, and it is spreading like wildfire. I also believe that it is being down-played so as not to cause a panic. Wake up, America!

Almost every aspect of the body's defenses can be compromised by generalized malnutrition. Individual nutrients affect immune response. Deficiencies of some nutrients can affect the tissue barriers against infection. Nutrient deficiencies also can alter immune systems that are controlled at the cellular level. They can inhibit the formation of antibodies, impair production of other infection-fighting substances, and cause other problems. Inadequate vitamin E will depress general host resistance. However, megadoses can inhibit several immune functions. Deficits as well as excessive supplies of both iron and zinc can be immunosuppressive. So take care not to abuse nutritional supplements.

Many cancers could be prevented by reducing our exposure to carcinogens. Some carcinogens can be avoided by personal choice. Reducing or avoiding exposure to cancer-causing agents can help to lower cancer rates.

Cancers develop slowly, usually appearing five or more years after exposure to a cancer causing agent. This long latent period is one reason why it is so difficult to identify the causes of human cancer. Many people exposed to a cancer-causing agent never develop cancer. Cancer of the lungs, for example, may not appear until thirty years after exposure to tobacco smoke or asbestos. This long delay can also happen with liver cancer after exposure to vinyl chloride, or bladder cancer after exposure to benzine or sodium saccharin.

Some carcinogens and other environmental factors are a direct cause of cancer, by causing the changes that turn a normal cell into a cancer cell. Other factors can act as indirect causes, by setting up conditions that help the action of other causes. We are dealing mainly with chemical carcinogens.

Human cancers have occurred following very low-level exposure. Asbestos brought home on the clothing of asbestos workers, for example, has caused fatal cancers in members of the workers' families.

A low exposure that might be safe for one person might cause cancer in another. Each person's individual environment and life-style can be a part of this variation. For example, a worker exposed to asbestos will be much more likely to develop lung cancer if he or she smokes.

Unfortunately, scientists have not yet developed a way to measure a person's individual risk. Exposure to a low level of a carcinogen thus has to be considered a risk for everyone. Studies have shown greater jumps in cancer rates from multiple exposures.

Tests on animals can identify substances that are likely' to be human carcinogens. Mice or rats are most commonly used for such tests because they are small, easily handled, more economical than larger animals, and generally similar to humans in their response to carcinogens. Most major forms of human cancer have been reproduced in such animals through exposure to chemical carcinogens. Since their natural lifetime is two to three years, rodents generally provide information about the cancer-causing potential of the test materials more quickly than do longer-lived animals, such as dogs or monkeys. Special strains of mice and rats have been used, and they have been responsible for saving millions of lives over the years.

There are self-righteous groups that are against using these animals for testing in this manner. I have one thing to ask them. How would they feel about it if one of their loved ones came down with a deadly disease, and their cure depended on tests that had to be carried out on an animal? I think I know the answer. Human life is much more important than rats' lives, in my opinion. Also, considering the number of lives saved by a handful of animals that gave their lives in the tests, there is no question in my mind that human life *is* more important.

Direct human exposures to cancer-causing substances often occur, and we can study the exposed populations. For example, people who have been exposed to tobacco smoke or asbestos develop a higher frequency of cancer of the lungs and other organs than unexposed people. From such population studies we have identified about thirty agents or industrial processes as causes of human cancers. Here is a list of causes along with examples of ways people can be exposed to them or might have been exposed in the past.

CAUSE	EXPOSURE
4-Aminobiphenyl	Antioxidant in rubber, manufacture of dyes
Arsenic and inorganic arsenic compounds.	Pesticides, manufacture of

arsenic compounds	glass and ceramics, smelting of metal ores, processed foods
Asbestos	Manufacture of asbestos-containing insulation. Break linings
Auramine	Manufacture of dyes
Benzene	Manufacture of chemicals and plastics, paints and adhesives, gasoline fumes
Benzidine	Manufacture of dyes
N,N-Bis- (2-chloroethyl)-	Drugs
2- napthylamine Bis (chloromethyl) Ether	Manufacture of chemicals and plastics
Cadmium and cadmium compounds	Electroplating, manufacture of metal alloys and batteries, inks and artists' colors, processed foods
Chloromethyl methyl ether	Manufacture of chemicals and plastics
Cromium and chromium compounds	Manufacture of metal alloys and protective coating on metals, paint, processed food
Cyclophosphamide	Drugs
Diethylstilbestrol	Drugs

Hematite and iron oxide	Mining of iron ore
Isopropyl oils	Manufacture of isopropyl alcohol
Melphalan	Drug
Mustard gas	Chemical warfare agent
2-Naphthylamine	Manufacture of dyes
Nickel and nickel compounds	Manufacture of metal alloys and metal plating, paint, and processed food
Oxymetholone	Drug
Phenacetin	Drug
Phenytoin sodium and Phenytoin	Drug
Radiation and radioactive materials	Sunlight, medical exams, industrial processes
Soots, tars, and oils	Manufacture of coal tar and creosote crude mineral oils and cutting oils
Tobacco and tobacco smoke	Cigarette, cigars and snuff
Vinyl chloride	Manufacture of plastics

The chemical used in the decaffeination process causes cancer. There is clear evidence of carcinogenicity of the chemical called methylene chloride that is used by coffee companies to decaffeinate coffee products. Most major American coffee decaffeinators rely on the the less expensive chemical methylene chloride, even though they are aware of the risk to human life, rather than using the harmless although more expensive method of steam-water process.

The companies abandoned another highly toxic chemical they were using called trichlorethylene when the FDA took action and banned it. The chemical methylene chloride is used widely in industry as a solvent in paint removers, as a degreasing agent, and in the manufacture of steroids, antibodies and other uses.

The study of methylene chloride found "clear evidence of carcinogenicity" in male and female mice as shown by increased incidences of lung growths. The phrase "clear evidence of carcinogencity" is the strongest language used by the National Toxicology Program in interpretations of animal studies. (The categories are "clear evident," "equivocal evidence," "no evidence" and "inadequate study.")

Some coffee makers denied using the chemical, however it was found while testing. While coffee makers are not required to report how they decaffeinate by the FDA, growing public concern about the decaffeination process has prompted a number of large companies to promote their products as "naturally decaffeinated." Others stand by the use of methylene chloride.

The chemical methylene chloride is toxic to the lungs if inhaled. This is only the fumes. Ingesting it is even worse.

This is another good example of the importance of reading the labels on the products we buy to consume.

My grandmother summed it up one day. She never trusted the chemicals used in the decaffeination process. She always said "I would rather have a little bit of caffeine that I get in the two cups of coffee I drink a day, than to have all that methylene chloride, or trichlorethylene that I would get in decaffeinated coffee." And I agree with her. If we keep our consumption of coffee down to two or three cups a day, the small amount of caffeine we would get would not be harmful to our bodies.

We must remember, too, that there are other products that contain caffeine, including soft drinks and some candies.

So again, be aware of what you are eating and drinking, and remember that it is important to use moderation in everything we do. It will keep us healthy, and also give us peace of mind.

You know, even if someday, happily, a cure for cancer is found, the effects of these chemicals, pesticides and additives in our diets will still destroy our livers, kidneys, bladders, and most of all, our immune systems. So we shouldn't count on a cure for cancer to solve all our problems. Let's take good care of our health, and make our bodies strong, so we won't need a "magic bullet," even if it is there for us.

Chapter 13

Food Additives and Pesticides

There was an amendment the Food, Drug, and Cosmetic Act in 1958 called the Delaney Clause. The amendment contains this brief paragraph: "No additive shall be deemed to be safe if it is found to induce cancer when ingested by man or animal, or if it is found, after tests that are appropriate for the evaluation of the safety of food additives, to induce cancer in man or animal." Yet, there are many foods on the shelves of supermarkets today with these same additives, which cause cancer.

We should all become informed and learn what the various additives are and what they do in our food. Read labels to find out what is in the foods you are buying. Select foods on the basis of what is good for you, not on convenience, appeal, color, or storage-time. The main reason the manufacturer puts additives and preservatives in food is to obtain longer shelf life so they can make more money and not have to deliver their products as often. They are not at all concerned with the effects of the additives on our health. We should make our views known. Let manufacturers know what you want and don't want in your food. Their name and address appears on each food label.

I don't believe God meant for a loaf of bread to last for two or three months. This is how long a loaf of bread sometimes lasts when they put calcium propionate in it to prevent mold. I'm sure after a week or two, most of the nutrients are gone. One day I was visiting a friend who was cleaning her kitchen, and found a small loaf of rye bread that had fallen down behind her refrigerator, where she had stacked several loaves, while preparing for a dinner party about six months previously. She opened it up, and other than being a little hard, it looked pretty good. We read the label, and sure enough, there were enough preservatives to choke a horse.

The Food and Drug Adminstration has been putting off decisions on banning artificial colors, which have been found to cause cancer in animals. It has postponed action since the proposal was first made in 1960. A decision to ban sulfites has been pending at the FDA since 1982. A ban on antibiotics in animal feed was first proposed in 1977 and action on it is still pending. The antibiotics are being fed to the animals, and the public eats the animal meat. All the antibiotics go into the human system, and I believe they have an accumulative effect on our bodies. I also believe this same thing happens when the animals are fed hormones. I believe our bodies are a living trash can for all the drugs that are fed to livestock, and we, the American people are paying for it with our lives. I believe the FDA should ban the drug sulfamethazine from our food supply. Sulfamethazine causes cancerous tumors of the thyroid glands, and also the thymus glands of animals. The thymus gland plays an important part in the immune system. The drug sulfamethazine is being given to animals, and when we eat the meat, or drink the milk, it goes into our bodies, remains there, and destroys our immune system.

The FDA recently banned the drug-preservative sulfite compounds, however, the manufacturers are still adding sodium sulfite, sodium bisulfite, sodium metabisulfite and potassium metabisulfite to our foods. The chemicals can be found in canned, dehydrated, and frozen foods. Also dried light-colored fruits, fruit juices, purees and fillings, maraschino cherries, gelatin, potatoes (including fresh-cut, dried, frozen, or canned), dry salad dressing mix, relishes, canned and dried gravies, sauerkraut, canned or dried shrimp or lobster soups, dried cod, frozen, canned, or dried vegetables, wine vinegar and baked goods. We still need to check ingredients lists carefully for the presence of these additives, which are poisoning our livers, kidneys and thymus glands, and actually killing people. The latest I have heard about is a ten-year-old girl from Oregon who consumed guacamole that was later found to contain high levels of sulfite preservative.

I believe the answer to this problem, since the FDA is dragging its feet on this issue, is to boycott every product that contains sulfite substances including sulfur dioxide, sodium sulfite, sodium and potassium bisulfite and sodium and potassium metabisulfite. If we all get together and boycott all these products, and the manufacturers are left with all these millions of dollars worth of products on their hands, that no one will buy, it will send a message loud and clear, that we are not going to take it anymore. It will get them in the pocketbook where it hurts the most, and they will be forced to give us good wholesome food again.

This is what happened with the pesticide Alar, which was being sprayed on apples. When everyone stopped buying apples, and they were rotting in the warehouses, the growers certainly got the message. And if you remember, the growers didn't waste any time cutting out the application of daminizide (Alar) on the apples. This show of unity and strength is what it takes to get our message across to them—we are not going to sit quietly by, while they poison our systems with their preservatives, chemicals, additives, and pesticides!

Speaking of pesticides, there are a few ideas I have about them, that I would like to share with you.

The wax from honeybees is not harmful in itself. However, the wax that the producers apply to fresh fruits and vegetables to make them shiny and attractive, seals in the pesticides that are on the outside of the fruit and vegetables making it impossible to wash off, you have to cut it off. Also they are not using pure beeswax. They are using shellac! And polyethlene! Can you imagine what effect this can have on your immune system? So be sure that you cut the peeling off of apples, pears, plums, and most of all, peaches. The fuzzy covering tends to hold more pesticides than a smoother surfaced fruit. And don't forget vegetables. The beautiful green outer peeling is so nutritious, on cucumbers and squash et cetera. However, if it is not homegrown, use the potato peeler, and peel the outer layer, which contains the pesticides and wax, off of it. Do the same with carrots, potatoes, and everything else that you feel has pesticides on it that you can't wash off. The packing plants use a combination of waxes, including shellac, carnuba wax, polyethlene and paraffin-type waxes—even on tomatoes, strawberries and bell peppers.

The insecticide ethyl paranitrolphenyl thiobenzene phosphonate which is put on almonds and walnuts in the amount of five hundred parts per billion and on apples, cherries, and citrus fruits in the amount of three thousand parts per billion is shocking. The herbicide Fusilade was approved by the Environmental Protection Agency (EPA), even though it caused birth defects in rats.

When different pesticides are used together, they are fifty percent stronger than if they are used individually. For example, when the pesticides malathion and EPTP (ethyl paranitrolphenyl thiobenzene phosphonate) are fed to lab animals, the combined effect is fifty times greater than the sum of their individual effects.

So how do we know what chemicals we are eating, how much we are eating, and in what combinations? We don't. All we can do it try to avoid them. Wash those vegetables and fruits, and remove all the outer peelings. Buy domestic grown foods. Boycott all foods that have the pesticides on them. Try to find small farms in the outlying regions.

If you buy from so-called organic food stores, be sure and check them out. Some are very deceptive. Ask them where the produce comes from. If they are not forthright, or hesitate or refuse to answer your question, go elsewhere.

When the big apple scare came up, there was a store in Beverly Hills that advertised apples that were organically grown, and had no Alar on them. However, when the apples were tested, they were found to have great amounts of Alar residue. Even after the evidence was shown to the store owner, she denied it.

My grandmother would go out to the country to buy most of her produce. She knew some elderly farmers out there where she would get fresh milk, eggs, and tons of fresh fruit and vegetables, for her patients who lived upstairs in her home. These farmers never used any pesticides on their produce. However it is very difficult to find a small farmer anymore, because of the economic difficulties facing them. Many are financially strapped, and are facing ruin because of the glut of foreign foods on the market. A strong dollar and weak tariffs do not help the situation. We should give local foods a chance, and not buy imports because they seem more exotic, or are a few cents cheaper. We should not only pay attention to the ingredients on packaged foods, but to the origin of all foods sold in today's markets. You have every right to ask: Is this a domestic tomato? Where are these grapes from? The disappearance of the family farm will be a sad chapter in our history. Let's try to keep them functioning as long as possible.

Another reason to buy domestic grown foods, is because our country (although there is a lot left to be desired) at least tries to control the amounts and kinds of pesticides used. Other countries, especially Mexico, have no standards at all. The boxes of poisons and pesticides have a warning label on them, because they are made in the United States. However the little children that they get to spray on the pesticides (most of whom cannot read at all, let alone read English) are unaware of the danger. The labels clearly state: "Do not let this liquid contact the skin." The young boys are out there barefoot, with the pesticides running down their arms and legs, and walking in it. After a while, I read, the young boys get very ill and some of them die. And the worst part of it is the doctors that examine them, don't know what was causing this. So it continues on and on.

Because of this situation in Mexico, I never buy produce that is grown there. We must do everything we can to protect ourselves from all the pesticides, the broad term the officials use for insecticides, herbicides, fungicides and other chemicals used to combat pests.

Environmentalists, scientists and other experts agree that the threat of pesticides to public health and the environment had increased the last quarter century, and that something must be done about it right away. The government has so far failed to carry out Congress's mandate of 1972 to protect people and the land, air, water, and wildlife from the chemicals. The experts say it may be well into the next century before all the dangerous pesticides are banned, restricted, or regulated.

The risks from pesticides are so much greater because of the exposures involved. Toxic waste dumps may affect a few thousand people who live around them. But virtually everyone is exposed to pesticides. A number of developments in recent years have added new urgency to the need to regulate pesticides, experts say. They have discovered that pesticides appear in underground water supplies despite an earlier belief that they would not pass through the soil. Today seventeen pesticides, including aldicarb and ethylene dibromide, either of which might cause cancer in humans, have been found in the ground water of twenty-three states.

They have discovered that some poisons registered for use in the fifties, sixties, and seventies can cause cancer, mutuations, and birth defects in humans. For most of the other chemicals on the market there is insufficient and sometimes fraudulently reported information about their effects on health and the environment.

They have discovered pesticide residue in a growing number of food products.

There is growing awareness that huge volumes of pesticides are used inside homes, factories, and hospitals, and on lawns and farms, often by people untrained in their use or unaware of their dangers.

There are complaints that farm workers are still inadequately protected from pesticides and that widespread illness results.

There is a growing export of pesticides, some of which are banned in this country, to developing countries where they often are uncontrolled.

Over twelve years after it was banned, the potent pesticide DDT persists in soil throughout the state of California, and detectable (but reportedly safe) levels are continuing to show up in vegetables, the state Department of Food and Agriculture said. It is very difficult to get evidence that DDT is being used illegally, but it is suspected. DDT was detected in crops in which an edible portion grows in, or close to, the ground, such as carrots, beets, lettuce and spinach. In a year-long study ordered by the Assembly, in part because of suspicions of illegal use of DDT by some growers, the department found widespread DDT levels throughout California's principal agricultural areas. The report said DDT was detected in all ninety-nine soil samples taken in thirty-two counties. The department concluded that half of the DDT used before it was prohibited at the end of 1972 is still in the environment. Therefore if there is continued use of it even though illegal, it will remain in California soil for at least another twenty or thirty years.

We must not forget the legacy of long-term, widespread environmental contamination that the use of DDT has left us, and will continue to leave us if this clandestine use of this poison is continued.

Like many of the other pesticides, DDT principally accumulated in the fatty tissues of fish and animals that have eaten it in feed and grain, and stays there forever, to be in turn eaten by humans in the meat of the animal, and the milk that we drink.

There is a DDT substitute known as dicofol that is possibly adding new levels of DDT to the environment. The level of DDT in dicofol is at least ten percent before it is formulated into commercial pesticides. Dicofol is used on cotton, fruits and vegetables, as well as lawns. DDT is still widely used in developing countries (another reason to try to buy domestic produce).

Many officials believe that we are consuming large and harmful amounts of pesticide residues. However any residue, no matter how little or how legal, is harmful. I believe that the government system to assure meat is free of dangerous chemicals has broken down. Predictable inspections and ineffective follow-up methods hamper federal efforts to detect chemical contamination, trace it back to its source and determine toxicity. The hormones injected into cattle are also worrisome. These hormones have been known to stay in the body, accumulating and causing problems with the immune system.

Chapter 14

Antibiotics in Our Food

At least ninety percent of this nation's swine and cattle are fed antibiotics, and virtually all poultry also ingest the drugs. Scientists say that the widespread practice of adding antibiotics to the feed of livestock and poultry to fatten the animals is dangerous. Humans are falling prey to especially virulent forms of diseases. The FDA should ban the use of penicillin and tetracycline in animal food. Producers are adding these drugs to the feed of the animals, so that the animals will get fatter faster, and they can get them to market sooner. Antibiotics, which are added to the feed also make possible the intense crowding of animals in the modern "factory farms" that dominate American agriculture and allow producers to benefit from it in dollars. They are making more and more money, with no concern whatsoever for the risk to human lives. These same producers certainly do not eat this same beef, or drink this milk that comes from the drugged cattle. No sir. They have their own private ranches, where the cattle are only fed pure grains and feed. They certainly are not going to risk their lives, and the lives of their families.

Manufacturing antibiotics for animal feed is big business. About half of the thirty-five million pounds of antibiotics produced in the United States every year go into animal feed. The annual bill for the animal antibiotics is $250 million.

The federal Center for Disease Control traced an outbreak of salmonella poisoning in eighteen people in four midwestern states to hamburger made from cattle that had been fed tetracycline on a South Dakota farm. They concluded the drugs had wiped out the victims' protective bacteria.

Several strains of bacteria that affect humans have already become alarmingly resistant to drugs. Eighty percent of the organisms that cause strep throat do not respond to the tetracycline any longer, twenty-five percent of the salmonella strains, which cause gastrointestinal illnesses, are unfazed by ampicillin.

Some researchers believe that the practice of feeding antibiotics to animals is causing a serious health threat to the human body. They believe it will create strains of super bacteria in meat-producing animals that will prove resistant to treatment. Consequently, the meat will carry these drug-resistant bacteria to humans.

The Center for Science in the Public Interest claims that antibiotic-laced animal feed is responsible for 270,000 cases of salmonella infection in humans and over 100 deaths each year.

Cash stimulates gluttony. In order to make more money, these producers of meat and milk are risking our lives, and we have to do something about it. We can start by hitting them where it hurts the most, in their pocketbook. If we all boycott these foods for only a few weeks, the companies will get the message, and they won't waste any time cutting out the antibiotics in the feed they give to the cattle. The loss of sales for this long, nationwide, will result in a great amount of money lost, and the contaminated food will have to be thrown away.

If the antibiotics in the cattle feed is not enough, add to that the injection of a chemical called diethylstilbestrol, into the cattle. Commonly known as DES, it is a synthetic hormone that acts like the female sex hormone estrogen. DES is used as a growth stimulant for cattle. Residues of DES have been found in meat and liver, from DES treated animals.

DES also causes cancer in people. Cancers of the vagina and cervix have developed in young women whose mothers were treated with DES during pregnancy. DES is a carcinogen when consumed, and such carcinogens cannot be added, intentionally or accidentally, to human foods. So why are they adding it to the cattle? To make the cattle fatter faster. More big bucks.

Also add to this the nitrates and nitrites that are being used to cure these same meats. Nitrates and nitrites are primarily used for coloring and flavoring. They give hot dogs, cold cuts, and ham their characteristic pink color. Without these additives, these meats would have brownish or grayish hue, like bratwurst. Is the pink color worth the risk? No! Nitrates can be changed by digestive juices into nitrites and nitrites can combine with other foods substances called amines to form nitrosamines. Nitrosamines can form in nitrite-treated foods before cooking and as a result of cooking at high temperatures. They also form in the acid stomach of laboratory animals, and in human beings as well. They are among the most potent cancer-causing substances yet discovered and readily induce several different types of cancers in virtually all species of laboratory animals. I believe that sodium nitrate should be banned from our foods. And we should use sodium ascorbate (a form of vitamin C) to block the formation of nitrosamines.

If you want to avoid needless exposure to nitrates and nitrites, start reading the labels, and boycott all products that are prepared with them. Better yet, limit your consumption of these foods, because they are all heavily laden with saturated fats and cholesterol.

Getting back to the color of the foods we eat, I must touch on the subject of food coloring. This is a controversial additive that is being used to make our foods look better, at the risk of our health. Because their purpose is purely cosmetic, even the slightest risk associated with their use is too great.

In the past half century more than a dozen food colors made from coal tar have been banned because they were found to damage internal organs or cause cancer. Too late for some people. Why don't they test these additives before they give them to us to eat? And then, if they are safe, go ahead and add them to our foods. What are we anyway, guinea pigs?

Citrus red dye no. 2 can be used to dye the outer skin of oranges, but then they use the orange peeling for marmalade, so we are still getting it in our diets. The same with yellow dye no. 5. It is still being used. More than 25 percent of the foods Americans eat are artifically colored. There is good reason to fight these synthetic food colors as well as all other poisonous foods additives. But the least we can do is not buy the factory-processed junk foods.

If we all stopped buying these foods, they would soon disappear from the grocer's shelves, and be replaced with good wholesome foods.

When I started writing this book, my intention was not to be critical of anyone. Because it is easy to sit back and criticize something or someone. What I'm trying very hard to do is find some solutions to some of our problems here in the United States. And to try to obtain the answers to questions and problems in order to help make this wonderful land where we live a safer place, with a healthier environment.

Now looking back, I find I have been very critical of some of the agencies and institutions that are in charge of our health and welfare. However I believe the criticism is well placed, since we all place our faith, health, and our very lives in their hands. We place our trust and our blind faith with a few people at the top to make the decisions that will affect our health and our very lives, because that is the American way. And compared to a lot of other countries, it is a good way, but I believe we can and should make it better.

I have written to many of our politicians about my doubts

and my concerns. I have not yet received any replies, but I believe that if we all get together, and write more letters, and boycott all the products that contain poisonous additives, articifical preservatives, antibiotics, pesticides, herbicides, poisonous chemicals and hormones, at least we will know that we have done everything possible to protect ourselves. It is not possible to eliminate all that is bad in our diets. However, if we are aware, and cut out most of the bad things, and see to it that we get our important nutrition, we will be much healthier and we will definitely live longer and happier lives.

It seems to me there is a monetary factor here. Taking into consideration the recent reports of influential people being convicted of accepting bribes, lying to the U.S. Congress, insider trading in the stock market, tax evasion, and even on the level of the people in the ministry, whom we should be able to trust the most, the discovery of "bad judgment" and "greed," I am convinced of this possibility.

Why should these producers of meat discontinue the use of hormones, antibiotics, and chemicals when they are making so much money? Why should the manufacturers stop using additives and preservatives, when they are saving so much money? Why should the farmers stop using the pesticides, herbicides, and chemicals, when they are making so much money? All the while, these influential executives of these big companies are aware of the obvious danger and threat to our health and our very lives. It is so clear, that they are nonchalant and unconcerned about the public's health and lives.

Even the most unsophisticated and impoverished citizens of this Southern California area, are aware of the misuse of these chemicals on and in our produce and processed foods. I have talked to many of the workers in the fields and in the factories. They are very much aware of the violations and the misuse of poisonous chemicals. However they are reluctant to come forward, because of the intimidation of their superiors and supervisors. The executives of the producers and the manufacturers must be held to account for this situation, because to be unaware of the situation, they would have to have a paper bag over their heads, or be blind, take your choice, I am convinced that they know exactly what they are doing. The reason I believe is money. I can't think of any other reason for them to risk the lives of all the American people by adding poison to the foods we eat. If you, the reader, have any opinions on the subject, I would really appreciate a letter on the subject. If I am ever wrong, I will be the first to admit it.

If you wish to write, please send your letter to the publisher and your correspondence will be forwarded to me. I will personally answer every letter. We are all at risk, and we are all in the same boat. So we should all get together and try to put an end to this poisoning of America.

I would donate to any committee, and give freely of my time to anyone that would start an investigation to find out what's going on and find some solutions to these life-threatening problems.

I would be very happy and grateful to hear from anyone who is interested.

Chapter 15

We Must Fight for Food Safety

There is the beginning of a crisis in the confidence of food safety today, and we should all get on the bandwagon and let our voices be heard. We should all get on the wave, and it will turn the tide, in the fight against pesticides. Once the farmers know that we are serious about it, and they start losing money because of produce staying on the shelf too long, because no one will buy it, then they will be forced to make changes in their methods.

About five percent of the nation's 2.1 million farmers have already adopted some form of alternative agricultural technology. There are sometimes new, sometimes old, practices that can improve the ecology and the economics of farming. We have real opportunities to improve the quality of the food supply and there is no need to make a trade-off on the protection of the environment. The only ones against this alternative are the manufacturers of fertilizer and other farm chemicals. They can see the golden goose going down the drain.

Some studies have cited numerous examples of how new methods of environmentally sound farming are succeeding. These include crop rotation, certain soil conservation practices, reductions in pesticide use and increased use of the biological and cultural means of pest control. Changing public opinion on this issue will provide the economic incentive for farmers to explore ways of reducing residues in food and the environment, because the demand for such foods will expand.

One more thing that concerns the little people, like us, is the notion that we have to buy picture-perfect produce. A big part of using the pesticides is because we desire cosmetically perfect produce. Cosmetic standards often have no relation to nutritional quality, flavor, or food safety. Pesticides applied solely to meet cosmetic standards increase residues of pesticides in food and hazards to agricultural workers. If I knew that I could buy clean, pesticide-free produce, I wouldn't mind if I found a blemish or two (that I could easily cut off) here and there. If they would stop using the chemical dyes that are so hazardous to our health, I wouldn't mind buying an apple that was not quite as red as before, or an orange that was not quite as orange in color as before. We don't need the cosmetic standards as much as we need clean, wholesome produce.

Progress could be amazingly brisk if economic incentives become available. The American food industry has demonstrated over the years incredible ingenuity and resiliency.

In 1951, Doctor Fred warned everyone about DES, the hormone used to artifically stimulate growth in animals. Twenty years later the FDA banned its use because it is a deadly carcinogen.

In 1952, Doctor Fred warned everyone about DDT in our food. Twenty years later it was banned.

In 1954, Doctor Fred warned everyone about the danger of cyclamates. It took them fifteen years to ban them. However, after all these years, these chemicals are still being used. And they can be found in the top soil of much of the land. It will take many more years for these poisons to dissipate.

If each one of us would write a letter to the presidents of the big food chains in our area, and let them know how we feel about pesticides, and state that we cannot continue to purchase these products containing them, it would make a big difference. There would be some drastic changes quickly. We must hit them in the pocketbook in order to get their attention. If you like, you may write to me, and I will see to it that the proper people receive all the letters. Let them know that reports like the one that came out in the middle of March of 1989 surrounding pesticides, that recommended daily consumption of at least five servings of produce in order to reduce the risk of cancer. And that "the benefits of such a diet in terms of a reduced risk of lung, stomach, and colon cancer far outweighted the risk an individual would receive from pesticide residues," are either trying to cover up or at least ignore the fact that the pesticides are on our produce, and any amount of pesticides no matter how small, are dangerous and will not be tolerated.

Mention the food additives and preservatives. Let them know that preservatives like sodium nitrite and sodium nitrate are no longer acceptable. Also tell them to stop using dyes such as yellow dye #5 (tartrazine). Our systems can do without all those dyes. Let them know that we can learn to appreciate the natural colors of good wholesome food.

When word got out this year that use of daminozide (trade name, Alar) was threatening the safety of apples, consumers were shaken and for good reason. If apples, our national fruit, and famous for healthy eating, could not be trusted, what was going on down on the farm? In their desire to produce larger and more abundant crops, they were putting the public and the environment at risk.

For years, Doctor Fred warned us about the dangers of all these chemicals and poisons. She recognized the need to find ways to grow food safely, and without further damage to the environment. Although conflicts do exist, farmers, environmentalists and consumers should find some common ground. We must question the methods of traditional agriculture.

Take nitrates, widely used as fertilizer. It has been known that using excess amounts to maximize crop production was causing a buildup in ground water, the reservoir that lies within and beneath the soil. It also has been known that levels of pesticides in ground water are rising. Most pesticides currently in use are herbicides, which are sprayed onto the produce, and consequently onto the ground. They, too, seep through to the ground water. Not only are levels higher, but the contamination has spread far from where the pesticides were originally applied. What makes this worrisome is that once these chemicals are dissolved or suspended in our ground water, they are there to stay.

In most of nature, plants grow without pesticides and fertilizers, so one suggestion is to identify natural methods of controlling pests, making use of pesticides unnecessary, along with a reduced need for fertilizer. Crop residues ranging from tomato plants to corn husks can be plowed back into the soil to enrich it. And leguminous plants with nitrogen-fixing bacteria in their roots can be used to furnish the nitrogen that crops need.

Representatives of the large food retailers in Southern California are stating that, "Calming consumers' fears over pesticide residues in produce is the key to increasing sales of fresh fruit and vegetables in the coming decade." No mention was made of cutting down or eliminating the pesticides. Just "calming the fears" of the consumer. In other words, as I see it, they are saying, pesticides are okay, or there are such small amounts of pesticides in the produce that they won't hurt you, so don't worry about it. Well, I do worry about these pesticides. And I hope you do, too.

Public concern over pesticide residues in food reached record highs during 1989. And for good reason. One representative stated, "The only thing that can stop us from increasing produce sales in the 1990s is further problems with food safety. We have to emphasize to the public how healthy produce is." Not one word about the possibility of cutting back on the amounts or elimination of these pesticides. Each of the representatives indicated awareness of the farm chemical problems. One stated that he was training their people to "handle the food safety questions, because it is a big issue."

Only one retailer mentioned that although it is important to make sure store employees are briefed on controversial issues such as pesticides it could be dangerous to mislead customers. "Sorting out opinion from fact is important. But if we are passing on information to our customers, it had better be real close to accurate or you're going to be in for some real trouble down the road."

Another countered, "Just ignore the pesticide problem, and emphasize the fact that produce is good for them. That's how we will sell more produce." It seems clear to me, that the most important thing concerning these supermarket representatives, is higher produce sales, and making more money, certainly not the health and welfare of their customers. Not one of the group there had anything to say about getting to the root of the problem, or finding alternative methods of protecting our food supplies.

After sitting through that meeting, I have some real doubts. I now wonder about all the things I have read and heard about the pesticide problems. What can you believe? How can I believe all the statistics that are quoted by officials regarding the amounts of poisons the farmers are adding to our food? Three different officials have quoted three different percentages of malathion that had been sprayed on the apples. Whom do we believe? Personally I won't be happy until they stop using pesticides altogether. And I believe that if enough of us get together and protest, and refuse to buy these products, that they will come up with an alternative to these pesticides. I would rather pay higher prices and get pure clean produce that I know won't kill me, than what we have now.

It is a well-known fact that daminozide and dioxen are

pure poison, and lethal to human beings. Yet they are still in widespread use in the United States. There are many alternative options open to commercial agriculture. These range from cases where farmers have successfully reduced their use of chemicals to the more stringent organic farming process. Also among the methods studied was integrated pest management, a technique that employs predator insects to destroy only those bugs that pose a threat to crops. There are other ways to approach the problem of crop infestation beside spraying with chemicals. But if we sit silently by, and continue to buy and consume the produce as it is now, the farms will never change their methods. Why should they? They are making money hand over fist. They must be made aware that we are not going to take it anymore. We have to let them know in no uncertain terms, before they will change their methods.

Chapter 16

Danger to the Immune System

Pesticides destroy the immune system and leave us open to many different types of disease and infection, including AIDS.

Immunity is the most important word in the field of medicine, as far as contending with all the new viruses that are being brought into this country, added to the ones that we already have.

We need immunity boosters. We need immune systems that are very healthy. The immune system is a vast network composed of trillions of specialized blood cells. The system has two basic functions. To recognize potentially harmful invading germs, and to respond protectively.

When the invaders are bacteria, the immune system, aided by antibiotics, is usually well prepared. Bacteria either float freely in the bloodstream or hook onto the surface membrane of the body tissues or organs. As a bacterium tried to reproduce, drugs such as penicillin perforate the bacterial cell wall. As a result, the bacterium virtually explodes, and special immune-system cells called macrophages clean up the debris.

However viruses are tougher to beat, since antibiotics do not work against them. Certain other aspects of the immune system assume a greater role than they do in fighting bacteria.

Unlike bacteria, which mostly remain outside cells, viruses invade individual cells. A flu virus, for example, begins its assault by fusing with and then penetrating a healthy cell. Once inside, the virus can transform a healthy cell into a miniature virus factory, reprogramming it so it will manufacture thousands more viruses. Soon bloated, the host cell bursts, unleashing a new generation to infiltrate other cells.

Left unchecked, the viral onslaught can eventually cause death. But in healthy bodies, the intruders soon encounter macrophages, which gobble up germs and signal defensive T and B cells to join the fight. When victory is finally achieved, immunity to that specific virus has been gained. If the same virus should attack again in the future, the immune system will reach full force immediately. Invaders are defeated before they do any damage, done in by antibodies, proteins made by the B cells that bind to a specific virus and signal special cells to move in for the kill.

Some experts say that chronic stress, anxiety, depression, and grief all trigger the brain to release hormones and chemicals called neuropeptides, which seem to hamper certain immune-system cells. The most recent evidence suggests that a balanced diet, regular, moderate exercise and stress reduction can be beneficial.

We believe that diet evaluations are necessary to assure proper amounts of essential nutrients. We feel that extra vitamin C, E, and B-complex should be included in the diet. And that it is imperative to eliminate all chemicals, hormones, preservatives, and insecticides that are added to food products.

We feel that fish and oysters are very important to restore the health, and that the answer to most of our ills will come from the ocean, sometime in the near future. There is a whole world of wonderful things that will be discovered, that are in the depths of the beautiful seas.

In the meantime, we should try very hard to protect ourselves from the above mentioned poisons, eat healthy foods, and get up off our seats, and run around the block. And above all, we must think positively that we will survive.

The immune system is affected by many things. Diet is

important. A car will not run without gas and oil. And our bodies will not function properly without vitamins and minerals. We need extra vitamin C, E, B-complex and cod liver oil every day, along with fresh fruit, vegetables, eggs, oat-bran cereals, fish and oysters, milk and fruit juices including pineapple, grape, apple and grapefruit juice. And don't forget the broccoli.

Another important aspect is a positive attitude toward life. It is very important to be happy. We should count our blessings, and be happy with what we have, rather than dwell on the things we do not have. We can smile, for not only will it make someone else happy, it will make us feel good inside. And it is important to keep a good sense of humor. Next to love, humor is the best human emotion. Not only do people respond positively to a good-humored person, the person feels good, too. A smile doesn't cost anything, and it can brighten the day for at least two people. Humor relieves tension, and puts things in proper perspective. Laughing at ourselves can give us a feeling of well-being. Sharing a laugh with someone can strengthen a friendship. And a good laugh can boost our immune system.

We must learn to eliminate the stress in our lives. We must try not to worry so much, especially about those things that we have no control over.

It is never too late to start. Over fifty doesn't mean over the hill, even for people who have never exercised regularly. Despite years of sedentary living, it is still possible to become physically fit.

Try to tighten your muscles as you go about your everyday activities. If you are stuck in traffic, hold your feet an inch off the floorboard. Or at stoplights, don't let your feet touch the floorboard. This really tightens the leg and tummy muscles. If you are sitting at a desk, or any chair, keep your feet off the floor for short periods of time.

Another important tool for boosting the immune system is the mind. A positive attitude toward life, high self-esteem, faith, hope, and a good sense of humor will do wonders.

The mind controls the body and all of its functions. We must think ourselves well, if we are ill—and think ourselves tl if we are fat. If you are ill, of course go to the doctor, and take his advice, but help him along with your mind. Assume the positive attitude that you will get well. If you keep your faith, and hope, you will get well.

Self-esteem is also important. Remember that God never made any trash. All of us are important and beautiful in our own way.

Last but not least, is a good sense of humor. It's healthy to laugh and humor sparks creativity. Humor is not kids' stuff. Once I was chatting with a gentleman that is worth millions of dollars, and he told me that he always reads the comic page of the paper every day. He said he wouldn't miss this much needed humor in his busy day. A sense of humor helps you to take a step back from a problem that looks terrible up close. When the world is closing in, we have to do something to lighten the moment.

We should look for humor in reality and serious places, like newspapers and church bulletins.

We should all try to remember that when we are kind to another person, we are being kind to ourselves, too. And when we smile at someone, that smile reflects inward. Each one of us benefits from every smile, and every kind act that we give someone else. In making someone else happy, we are also making ourselves happy. So forget your troubles, and be happy.

Boosting our immune system is important, but many of us don't know how. We must keep it all our lives, because our immune system is our best friend. If we protect it, it will protect us.

Beta carotene, vitamins C and E are very important. Beta carotene can be found in carrots, spinach, sweet potatoes, winter squash, and cantaloupe. It is a nutrient that we need to protect us against cancer. It is one of a large group of substances called carotenoids, which are generally found in the same vegetables and fruits.

Unlike vitamin A, which can be very dangerous in large doses, beta carotene is nontoxic, since the body is able to regulate its conversion to vitamin A. The worst thing large amounts of carotene can do is turn the skin slightly yellow, but this is harmless. In addition, beta carotene comes from vegetable sources, which tend to be high in fiber as well as other carotenoids and lesser-known nutrients that are also protective. In contrast, vitamin A comes from animal sources.

Numerous animal studies have shown that beta carotene can defend against tumors and enhance the immune system. Many studies on humans have found that those who don't eat enough vegetables and fruits rich in carotenoids have an increased risk of cancer (lung cancer in particular). One recent large study found that people with low levels of beta carotene in the blood had a far higher risk of developing lung cancer as well as melanoma, a lethal form of skin cancer. Other carotenoids and nutrients in vegetables and fruits are also protective agents against cancer, and other diseases. Take the beautiful tomato for instance, a delicious vegetable.

The red globes are rich in a compound called lycopene that researchers have found lacking in people most apt to develop pancreatic cancer. The malignancy is especially virulent, killing 22,000 Americans yearly. The investigators examined blood samples collected ten years ago from 26,000 people. The scientists were searching for clues that might identify those likely to develop cancer of the pancreas.

Indeed, the cancer vicims' blood, compared with that of similar individuals who did not get cancer, showed one outstanding nutritional difference: low levels of a vegetable compound called lycopene. In fact, those with the least lycopene in their bloodstream had five times the chance of getting pancreatic cancer as those with the most blood lycopene.

Lycopene is a red pigment in fruits and vegetables, especially tomatoes and strawberries.

The researchers state that low blood levels of lycopene signified low consumption of such foods, and leaving pancreatic cells more vulnerable to damage. So let's eat our tomatoes every day.

Lycopene and beta carotene, like vitamins C and E, are antioxidants. That is, they seem to neutralize the free radicals that damage cells and contribute to cancer. In simplest terms, the way free radicals damage the body's cells is similar to the process by which oxygen causes paper to turn yellow or butter to turn rancid. Scientists believe that beta carotene and the other antioxidants each exert a protective effect at a different part of the cell and against different free radicals.

When we are shopping for food, we should look for orange, yellow, and dark green, the colors of vegetables and fruit that are rich in beta carotene. If we are like the average American, we should consume two to four times more carotene than we do now. A professor of food science says that people should eat foods supplying five to six milligrams of beta carotene a day.

A carrot a day along with our other fruits and vegetables, will do the job, and make sure that we get enough beta carotene, plus other important nutrients. A science report came out this year that confirms what Doctor Fred has always maintained. It recommended that Americans should eat at least five servings of various fruits and vegetables every day. But one survey showed that on any given day 50 percent of Americans eat only one vegetable, and 41 percent eat no fruit at all.

We are better off getting our beta carotene from foods than relying on carotene supplements, because not only will the foods give us additional nutrients that will play a role in protecting against cancer, the fruits and vegetables will give us more fiber. Which also helps in protection.

Frozen vegetables can retain as much carotene as fresh. However, cooking does destroy some carotene. The longer you cook, the more is destroyed. But we shouldn't cook vegetables long anyway. Rather undercook, than overcook, so as to preserve all the nutrients, including vitamin C.

Carrot Patch Pie is a heavenly way to get your quota of beta carotene.

4 eggs
1 cup milk
½ cup buttermilk baking mix
1 tablespoon minced onion

2 tablespoons lemon juice
1 teaspoon dillweed
1 teaspoon salt
1 package frozen sliced carrots or
10 ounces sliced fresh carrots,
cooked and drained
2 tablespoons sliced almonds

Reserving a few carrot slices for garnish, place all ingredients except almonds in blender, cover and blend at medium speed until smooth. About one minute. Carefully pour into well-coated (with margerine) nine inch pie plate. Bake in preheated 350 degree oven, for fifteen minutes. Remove from oven and sprinkle with almonds. Continue baking until puffy and knife inserted near center comes out clean, about another 15 to 20 minutes, drizzle margarine on top, and garnish with reserved carrot slices.

Eat soup to lose weight. Researchers found that a bowl of warm (not hot) soup at the start of a meal slows the rate of eating and fills the stomach, which signals the brain to curtail the appetite. My grandmother, Doctor Fred, would always recommend soup before a meal, when the patient needed to lose weight. Doctor Fred would also tell them not to keep cakes, cookies, doughnuts, pies and candy in the house. Just don't buy it. If it's not there you won't eat it. Buy fruit instead. An orange, apple, pear, or banana is sweet, filling, and much better for the body. You can eat pretty much the same foods that you usually eat, but by cutting out the sweet desserts, and cutting off all the fat from your steaks and pork chops, you will still lose weight. Also, cutting off all the fat from the meat is important, because most of the chemicals, pesticides, hormones and antibiotics that are given to the animals, are concentrated in the fat cells. And the animal fat goes straight to our hips and thighs.

Doctor Fred said not to give up eating eggs. Eggs are important to a healthy diet. We should include at least six eggs per week in our diets. The cholesterol in eggs is not harmful, if we eliminate the chemicals, preservatives, and additives in the food we eat, as I have outlined before.

There are other things we can do to cut out animal fats from our diets, to lose weight, and be healthier, too. Because if we eliminate the above-mentioned chemicals from our diets, our bodies will take care of the cholesterol, and assimilate it properly in the system. It is only if we assault our bodies with these poisons in our food, that they interfere with the proper elimination of HDL cholesterol. Here are a few healthy suggestions:

Steam, boil, or bake vegetables. Or stir-fry in small amount of vegetable oil.

Season vegetables with herbs and spices rather than butter.

Try lemon juice or apple-cider vinegar mixed with wheat germ oil on salads and vegetables.

Use margarine instead of butter in baked products, and use corn oil instead of shortening.

Try whole-grain flours to enhance flavors of baked goods, sauces, and gravies.

Replace whole milk with nonfat or lowfat milk in puddings, soups and baked goods.

Substitute plain lowfat or nonfat yogurt, blender-whipped lowfat cottage cheese and buttermilk and wheatgerm oil for sour cream dressing.

Choose lean, select cuts of meat and trim all the fat off, if you must have meat at all.

Remove skin from poultry before eating. And roast, bake, or broil rather than frying.

Cook meat or poultry on a rack so the fat will drain off, and use nonstick pan so added fat is unnecessary.

Chill broth until fat becomes solid, and spoon off fat before using the broth.

Remember that the body has to work harder to convert margarine and vegetable oil into fat than butter and animal fat. The butter and animal fat goes directly into the old spare tire.

We believe that pure fat that we consume from animals that have not been contaminated with chemicals, hormones, antibiotics, and pesticides will not cause the lesions in the arteries that cause heart attacks—as long as we are not getting these same chemicals, hormones, antibiotics, and pesticides from another source. In other words, we believe that the above-mentioned poisons that we consume every day in our diets, are responsible for interfering with the body's ability to properly assimilate the food, including fat, that we consume.

These poisons are also responsible for causing the buildup of fat in arteries, thus causing us to develop cardiovascular disease. This also explains why some of us develop this disease, and some of us do not. The more junk food with all the additives, preservatives, and color chemicals that we consume, the more likely we will be to develop this disease. Especially when we start eating these foods when we are young. The buildup of fat in the arteries, and the resulting lesions, start early. This is why it is so important to teach our children early in life to eat the proper foods, to avoid heart attacks at an early age.

If we can eliminate the above-mentioned poisons from our diets, we could enjoy all the good wholesome foods that our bodies need, like milk, eggs, butter, cheese, steaks, and pork chops, without worrying about heart attacks and cholesterol, because our bodies will take care of us.

If you have a beautiful expensive automobile, you would not go out and put sugar in the gas tank, would you? Of course not. Well you have a beautiful body, and please don't put chemicals, preservatives and pesticides in it. Remember, "You are what you eat."

Chapter 17

The Good Old Days

When I moved to California, I never dreamed that there was such a life-style difference from that on the ranch in Arizona. I found a whole new world. It was exciting, and yet very frightening.

When I was nine years old, I had to take care of livestock every morning and evening. I was in charge of taking the newborn calves, and teaching them how to drink milk from a pail. I had to get them to suck on my fingers, and then gently pull their heads down into the pail of milk, and wiggle my fingers around, so that milk would go up into the calf's mouth when he sucked on my fingers. Once I had him drinking the milk out of the pail, it was easy to feed him.

Every morning before school, and every evening after school, I had to feed all of the baby calves. They were so cute. When they saw me coming with my pails of milk, they would race to the gate, to get in line to be fed. I think they thought that I was their mother. Once they were full, they would go back into the alfalfa field, and play in the grass, or lie in the sun.

After a week on plain milk, I would start mixing calf meal in with the milk, along with vitamins and minerals. Each day the milk mixture would get thicker and thicker, until they finally were on solid food. By the time the calves were eating solid food, another herd of baby calves would come along, and I would start the cycle all over again. Those cows and calves were so healthy. There was never any antibiotics, hormones, or preservatives given to our cows or calves at any time of their lives. I never heard of these things. Things were different then. It makes me wonder about progress.

Another thing that we never ever used was pesticides. We, and all the rest of our neighbors got along just fine without any of the chemicals and poisons that the farmers use now. I believe it is time for America to wake up and smell the pesticides. We really don't need them. The pioneers that came to this land so long ago, and made it what it is, a beautiful country, never had pesticides, and chemicals and poisons. They never had preservatives. The only preservatives they had were natural ones like salt, pepper and spices. These wonderful people that worked so hard, and developed this land of ours ate beans, milk, butter, pure beef, and eggs. And I know of many who lived long and happy lives, never having heard of cholesterol.

I sincerely believe that we need cholesterol in our diets, and that the problem is with the action and interaction of the other things like chemicals, preservatives, additives, hormones, and pesticides that we put into our food and our bodies that interfere with the proper assimilation of some things including cholesterol. I believe that the healthy body that does not consume the above-mentioned chemicals, will properly regulate the HDL and LDL levels of cholesterol in the system. We must eliminate these chemicals from our diets, and give our bodies a chance to mend themselves—this means all our organs including the immune system—in order to be a properly functioning unit.

Our livers take a beating almost every day. Take for instance the bromides. Bromides are compounds derived from bromine, a chemical resembling cholorine. These chemicals are still being used by manufacturers even though they know the bromides should not be taken internally because they cause serious side effects including liver damage. We must not consume any bromides, period.

Yes, I do admit I long for the "good old days," when life

was carefree and uncomplicated. I remember when I was a child, the most complicated thing I had to worry about was the cream separator. I would stand for hours turning the handle of the separator. The cream would come out of one spout, and the milk would come out of another. The centrifugal force of the perforated cylinder would force the cream to the top spout, and the skim milk would pour out the bottom spout. I thought this was really interesting, and I was fascinated by how fast and easy the cream could be separated from the milk.

Little did I know what was ahead for me when I moved to the big city of Los Angeles only a few years later. And I was never really prepared for my first initiation into the hard reality of unscrupulous people.

I had come to Los Angeles to work my way through college. I had gone to California State, to check out the school and see if there were any job listings on the memo boards. I met a girl there, and we started talking. I told her that I had not found a place to live yet, and that I wanted to get a place near the college. Right away, she insisted that I come stay with her, and pay half of the rent. We also agreed that I would pay half of the utilities, which was fair. I was happy! I had been in town only two hours, and I already had a new friend, and a place to live. I was walking on air. This was the beginning of a beautiful life in sunny Southern California. She told me to follow her in my car.

When I got to her apartment. I hardly had my suitcases in the door, when she told me that since I would be paying half of the utilities, and that everything was due, so I should go down and pay everything now, and she would pay everything next month. With that, she handed me all the bills and the addresses, and then she asked me for the month's rent, also. I had not had a chance to open a checking account, so all I had was cash to give her. I gave her the rent, which was $450, and I went to pay her bills.

It took me quite a while, as I did not know my way around town. I finally took care of everything, and I went back to the apartment. When I returned there, I noticed that my suitcases were sitting outside the door. I knocked on the door, and the girl opened the peephole and asked me if I had paid all the utilities. I told her that I had, and I apologized for taking so long. I then asked her if I could come in. As I was standing in front of the door, I could see through the peephole, that there was a man standing behind her. The girl told me flatly that her boyfriend had come back from a trip, and that he would be staying there, and that I was not welcome there. I said, "What about the rent I paid you?" She said, "What about it?" I told her that since I could not stay there, that she should give me back my rent money, as I had little left, after paying her bills. She said, "Get lost!" I took my suitcases to my car, and put them in. With tears streaming down my face, I thanked God that she let me have my things back.

I sat there in my car wondering what to do next. I wanted to get out of there. I started driving, anywhere. I drove about a mile, and I was crying so hard that I decided to park for a while. I couldn't believe anyone could do anything like that. It was a nightmare. I had never felt so lost and alone before in my life. I also felt frightened and hurt.

After getting myself together, I drove to a residential neighborhood, parked the car, got out, and went to the door of a pretty home. There I found a nice lady, and I asked her if I could park in her driveway and sleep in my car for the night, as I had lost my money, and had no place to stay. The nice lady, God bless her, said it would be all right. I offered to give her the last of my money for the favor, but she declined.

Early the next morning, I heard a tapping on my window, and it was the lady and her sister, with a cup of hot coffee for me. I had never had coffee before, but I didn't tell them that. I just thanked them very much for their hospitality and drank that coffee. Those ladies, bless their hearts, gave me back some of my lost faith. And I will never forget them. I have tried so many times to remember where that house was, so I could take a small gift and thank them again, but since I was so upset when it happened, I forgot what street I was on. Since it was dark outside, I didn't even know what color the house was.

Well anyway, I proceeded to the main street to search for a service station, so I could use the restroom to wash my face and brush my teeth. I finally found a Union Oil Station, and they let me use their restroom. I was so grateful. Then I drove on for a while, and found a drive-in restaurant and went in to get a glass of milk. There was a terrific man there ranting and raving that one of his girls had not shown up for work, and he was having problems cooking and serving, too. Well I don't have to tell you, we worked out a deal very quickly that I would go to work for him right then. I would have worked for him just for my meals, at that point. However, he insisted on paying me, too. I worked for that man off and on for the next two years, between classes.

Then one day he told me that the lease had run out on the building, and he had to close up. I thanked him for all his kindness, and set out to find me another job.

The experience of the girl cheating me out of my money was a good lesson for me. At the time, I was so hurt, I thought it was the end of my life in California. But now looking back, and reading the newspaper about all the terrible things that happen to innocent girls, I realize I was very lucky that the only thing I lost was my money. It could have been much worse, I could have lost my car and or my life. So I am grateful that God spared me, and I did learn to be more careful about the people in whom I place my trust. I still can't believe that I was so dumb. But I was used to trusting everyone. The people that I grew up with were good hardworking, God-fearing, honest people.

Many years later I met a man that I fell head over heels in love with. He told me that he felt the same way about me. He said that he would like to spend the next thousand years with me. I was so happy. He was tall and very handsome but too thin. I thought that he needed someone to take care of him, and cook some good meals for him. And I wanted to be that someone.

When we had a date, it was hard for me to tell him goodnight. No matter how long we were together, it was never long enough. The time passed so quickly when we were together. And the time seemed endless when we were apart. When he came from work, he would stop in where I worked, because we worked different time shifts. I could hardly wait for him to walk in the door. I would watch for him, and when he walked in, my heart would almost stop. Yes, for the first time in my life, I was in love. Could I trust him? Could I believe the sweet things he told me? Would we spend the "next thousand years" together? Or would he break my heart and leave me to cry a million tears? Should I take the chance? (To be continued in my next book, "The End of the Rainbow.")